SO-AXW-848

The Secret to a
Long and
Healthy Life

Mother Nature's secret harvested from the sea contains everything you need to live a long and healthy life.

Dr. Eberhard Hartmann

THE NATIONAL HEALTH PRESS

More References and Clinical Studies
supporting the information and statements of this book

32. Krauss RM, Eckel RH, Howard B, Appel LJ, Daniels SR, Deckelbaum RJ, Erdman JW Jr. Kris-Etherton P, Goldberg IJ, Kotchen TA, Lichtenstein AH, Mitch WF, Mullis R, Robinson K, Wyhe-Rosett J, St Jeor S, Suttie J, Tribble OL, Bazzarre TL. *AHA Dietary Guidelines revision 2000: A statement for healthcare professionals from the Nutrition Committee of the American Heart Association.* Circulation. 2000; 102: 2284-2299.

33. Kris-Etherton PM, Harris WS, Appel LJ. for the Nutrition Committee. *Fish consumption, fish oil, omega-3 fatty acids, and cardiovascular disease.* Circulation, 2002; 106: 2747-57.

34. Lee TH, Mencia-Huerra JM, Shih C, Corey EJ, Lewis RA, Austen KF. *Effects of exogenous arachidonic, eicosapentaenoic and docosahexaenoic acids on the generation of 5-lipoxygenase pathway products by ionophore-activated human neutrophils.* J Clin Invest. 1984; 74: 1922-1933.

35. Maki KC, Reeves MS, Farmer M, Griinari M, Berge K, Vik H, Hubacher R, Rains TM. *Krill oil supplementation increases plasma concentrations of eicosapentaenoic and docosahexaenoic acids in overweight and obese men and women.* Nutr. Res. 2009; 29(9): 609-15.

36. McKenzie, J., *"Fish Oil Helps Treat Depression Study: Fish Oil Contains Natural Ingredients That Help Treat Depression",* ABC news, Aug.19. http://abcnews.go.com/WNT/MedicineCuttingEdge/.Story?id=1294988cpage=2

37. Mori TA, Woodman RJ, Burke V, Puddey IB, Croft KD, Beilin I.J. *Effect of eicosapentaenoic acid and docosahexaenoic acid on oxidative stress and inflammatory markers in treated-hypertensive type 2 diabetic subjects.* Free radic Biol Med. 2003; 35: 772-781.

38. Naguib YM. *Antioxidant activities of astaxanthine and related carotenoids.* I Agric Food Chem. 2000; 48: 1150-1154.

39. Niiveldt RJ, van Nood E, van Hoorn DE, Boelens PG, van Norren K, van Leeuwen PA. *Flavonoids: a review of probable mechanisms of action and potential applications.* Am J Clin Nutr. 2001; 74: 418-425.

40. Parra, D., et al., *"A diet rich in long chain omega-3 fatty acids modulates society in overweight and obese volunteers during weight loss",* Appetite Nov. 2008; 51(3): 676-80.

41. Paschos GK, Rallidis LS, Liakos GK, Panagiotakos D, Anastasiadis G, Votteas V, Zampelas A. *Background diet influences the anti-inflammatory effect of alpha-linolenic acid in dyslipidaemic subjects.* Br J Nutr. 2004; 92: 649-655.

42. Pischon T. Hankinson SE, Horamisligil GS, Rifal N, Willett WC, Rimm EB. *Habitual Dietary Intake of n-3 and n-6 Fatty acids in Relation to Inflammatory Markers Among US Men and women.* Circulation. 2003; 108: 155-160.

43. Priddy AR, Killick SR. *Eicosanoids and ovulation.* Prostaglandins Leukot Essent Fatty acids. 1993; 49: 827-831.

44. Sampalis F, Buena R, Pelland MF, Kowalski O, Duguet N, Dupuis S. *Evaluation of the effects of Neptune Krill Oil on the management of premenstrual syndrome and dysmenorrhea.* Altern Med Rev. 2003; 8(2): 171-9.

45. SanGiovanni, J., et al., *"The relationship of dietary omega-3 long chain polyunsaturated fatty acid intake with incident age-related macular degeneration: AREDS report no.23".* Arch. Ophtalmol. Sept. 2008; 126(9): 1,274-9.

46. Stall, A., et al., *"Omega 3 fatty acids in bipolar disorder: a preliminary double-blind, placebo-controlled trial,"* Arch. Gen. Psychiatry May 1999; 56(5): 407-12. Turnbull, T., et al., *"Efficacy of omega-3 fatty acid supplementation on improvement of bipolar symptoms: a systematic review, "* Arch. Psychiatr. Nuts. Oct. 2008; 22(5); 305-11.

47. Werner A, Havinga R, Kuipers F, Verkade HJ. *Treatment of EFA deficiency with dietary triglycerides or phospholipids in a murine model of extrahepatic cholestasis.* Am J Physiol Gastrointest Liver Physiol, 2004; 286: G822-G832.

48. Zamula, E., *"The Greenland Diet: Can fish oils prevent heart disease,"* FDA Consumer Oct. 1986; 20(8): 6-8.
   a. 11, 737 results based on "omega-3" search term at PubMed.gov, a service of the U.S. National Library of Medicine.
   b. *Helps on reduce serum triglycerides / triacylglycenols.* (Oh, 2005; Balk, et al., 2004; Hooper, et al., 2004; Nilsen, et al., 2001; Siatori, et al., 1998). Health Canada natural health products Directorate Monograph, Jan.10, 2008.
   c. *Helps support cognitive health and / or brain function* (I lag, 2003; Morris, et al. 2003; IOM, 2002). Health Canada Natural Products Directorate Monograph, Jan.10, 2008.
   d. *"Research Into Cardiovascular Benefits of Omega-3 Fatty Acids Highlighted By Mayo Clinic Proceedings,"* Medical News Today mar. 11, 2008; www.medicalnewstoday.com/articles/100175.php
   e. *"Fish oil outperforms statin in heart failure study,"* The Associated Press, Aug.31, 2008.
   f. *"Fish Oil".* Health Canada Natural Health Products Directorate Monograph, Jan.10, 2008.
   g. Study findings published in the medical journal *The Lancet* and announced at the European Society of Cardiology in Munich *International Herald Tribune* Aug. 31, 2008.

Foreword

Dear Reader,

I know many of you think hyperacidity and heartburn are just minor complaints. But did you know that hyperacidity (excess acid or acidosis) can actually make you ill?

Most of the food we eat such as meat, products made with white flour and even sweets and coffee are acidifiers. Consumed in too great a quantity, they acidify the fluids in the organism and make your body sick. You get "hyper-acidified". You feel ill, anxious, listless, tired and unmotivated, to name but only a few of the symptoms.

But the body has a defence mechanism against this type of excess acidity. It is designed to protect its cells against burning and destruction. Its strategy is to link excess acids to its stock of mineral salts (in other words, it neutralizes them) and store them as waste product. This in itself is already dangerous, but there's something else that's very worrying. Forced to combat this hyperacidity, the body needs increasing quantities of mineral salts and if your diet doesn't provide them, it digs in to its reserves, which results in demineralization. Linus Pauling, the Nobel prize-winning chemist said: *"Every disease is directly linked to a lack of mineral salts."*

Researchers have identified more than two hundred diseases that they believe are directly linked to a lack of mineral salts: diabetes, arthritis, heart disease, gallstones, kidney stones, along with many other illnesses. What this means is that the mineral salts we absorb through our regular diet is not enough to protect our health and so we should be taking mineral supplements as a result.

Since 1995, Doctor Grillo has been at the Artiga research station in Antarctica studying the beneficial effects of Krill on the animal organism. He noted that penguins, regardless of their age, never get any arteriosclerotic-type build up in their blood vessels, despite consuming enormous amounts of fat. He concluded that it must be due to their diet, which is essentially made up of Krill.

Krill is a Norwegian word, meaning "whale food". Krill forms the basis of the Antarctic ecosystem. It's the principle source of nutrition of whales, seals, icefishes, cuttlefish, penguins and albatrosses. It exists in enormous quantities. It's possible to extract precious nutrients from Krill, like the ones contained in the nutritional supplements of Antarctic Krill Oil soft gel capsules.

Antarctic Krill can be used in many different therapies. It's excellent for joint diseases (arthrosis, arthritis, rheumatism), cholesterol and basically any inflammatory disease. It works to relieve joint pain and can even be effective in treating cancers! In addition to all this, Antarctic Krill increases energy levels and boosts vitality.

Antarctic Krill is a product that comes directly to us from nature. Soft gel capsules of Antarctic Krill Oil, with the correct balance of carefully chosen ingredients, means that you can now have the natural marvel within your reach.

With my knowledge of the healthy benefits of Antarctic Krill, I've managed to pack everything you need to know on the subject in this small but essential book.

Today, it's easier to stay healthy than you might think. Now, you're going to make a completely natural discovery that is going to give you a new quality of life.

And that's what I wish for you, from the bottom of my heart.

Yours,

Dr. Eberhard Hartmann

CHAPTER 1
Always healthy and never sick – only a dream?

The perfect recipe from nature: How to prevent and cure excess acidity and inflammatory diseases

As I said earlier, one thing is certain, if there existed a magic formula that could help you achieve your dream of living in constant good health, without ever getting sick, it would have to contain some *very* special ingredients... But unfortunately, despite the constant advancement of modern medicine, eternal health will surely remain a dream forever. But a dream that 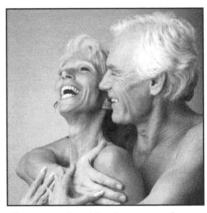 can teach us an important lesson: that you should take care of your health – all the time, for prevention as well as cure!

Health is a precious asset

These days, there's plenty that you can do to protect or stabilize your health. Many diseases that were completely incurable until only just a few years ago, can now be effectively treated, or at least controlled.

And though we know that progress can sometimes suffer setbacks, there's no denying that everyday medicine is taking ever greater strides towards combating disease.

Yes, Mother Nature has the cure...

In recent years, there has been a lot criticism towards medicine and the pharmaceutical industry by those who advocate a return to natural healing. Their arguments are simple and easy to understand: Human beings are creations of nature, so why wouldn't our diseases be cured with natural remedies? But even if, every week, we're discovering remedies found in nature that preserve health, promote well-being and strengthen both body and mind, there are still many

Americans who prefer to rely on all sorts of chemical drugs. And many need to take drugs simply to treat the adverse side-effects caused by the drugs they're taking to treat their condition! It's madness.

Yet, it's an indisputable fact: Mother Nature gives us everything we need to stay in good health.

Natural harmony

Let's dream a little and wonder how amazing it would be if there existed a natural remedy with the potential to cure your body, leaving your mind free to seek out new adventures and rise to new challenges. That would be really incredible, wouldn't it? You could reach your goal of living actively and in good health to a ripe old age, your body strong, never needing to undergo risky operations... Your mind and body in perfect harmony.

So, isn't it exciting to know there is already a way to achieve this, right here and now? All you need to do is figure out the causes of the many illnesses you suffer day in and day out and then identify an active ingredient, preferably natural, which cures them.

Fortunately, your dream may become reality sooner than you think! We have already discovered a natural active ingredient that works both to prevent and cure many different diseases. Let's learn more about this amazing secret in the following pages.

First, take this test:

Before we go on, can I ask you to take a few minutes – just a few minutes that could change your life – to answer the following questions honestly:

	YES	NO
• Do you often feel tired?	❏	❏
• Do you get heartburn, or have you had it in the past?	❏	❏
• Do you find yourself easily irritated?	❏	❏
• Do you suffer from joint pain, arthrosis, arthritis or rheumatism?	❏	❏
• Do you often feel down or overworked?	❏	❏
• Do you experience feelings of listlessness, fatigue, exhaustion and demotivation quite often?	❏	❏
• Do you get swellings?	❏	❏

	YES	NO
• Do you often suffer from bloating?	❏	❏
• Do you sometimes feel overwhelmed?	❏	❏
• Do you often suffer from anxiety?	❏	❏
• Do you get mood swings?	❏	❏
• Do you often get raging hunger pangs?	❏	❏
• Are you overweight?	❏	❏
• Do you sometimes get pain in your hands?	❏	❏
• When you get up in the morning, do you get pain in your joints or limbs?	❏	❏

Two more questions, for women:

	YES	NO
• Do you have painful periods (premenstrual syndrome)?	❏	❏
• Do you get pain, low down in your abdomen?	❏	❏

TOTAL _____

Test evaluation

If you answered YES at least 3 times to any of the questions above, then you absolutely must read the rest of this book. If you answered YES at least 6 times it's even more important and critical that you discover the information that is revealed to you in the next pages. These questions were geared towards identifying the symptoms of specific diseases.

If you continue reading, you are going to discover what is probably today, the most effective way to promote the healing process.

Now, you are now going to discover two conditions that are a major cause of a series of diseases.

Inflammatory disease and excess stomach acid

Perhaps these words don't mean very much to you. But as you are soon going to see, they are symptoms of many different diseases.

All of this is important to know, because it's the only way of determing the exact cure that is going to fight these diseases. Over the next few pages, let's discover how we can heal inflammatory diseases, effectively and from the inside.

You're also going to learn exactly why excess stomach acid is considered the primary cause of many conditions, why chronic disease often goes hand in hand with an acid base imbalance and you're going to learn why the lack of calcium and other mineral salts is responsible for many diseases.

How can we avoid these conditions and start protecting our health? That's what you're going to find out in the pages that follow!

Remember, heartburn can be a symptom, because:

Excess stomach acid is the Number 1 disease in the Western World today!

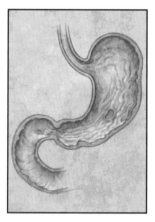

In recent years, there has been much talk in the media about "acid rain". But they fail to mention the fact that these same pollutants that are destroying our forests are also undermining our health creating a species of "acid beings". In North America, more than 91% of the population could be categorized as "acid beings".

Hyperacidity (excess stomach acid, acidosis) has become so widespread we tend to think it's unimportant. But, in the long-term, it's making us sick... very sick.

How is hyperacidity making you so sick?

Scientists have discovered that the organic liquids of a healthy person are alkaline (high pH), while those of a sick person are acidic (low pH). It's a fact that around 80% of the food you eat, such as meat, products made with white flour, and even desserts and coffee are acidifiers. In other words the body metabolizes them into acids. This means that only 20% of your diet is alkaline: fruits, vegetables, herbs and still water.

This would not, in itself, pose a serious problem, because the body strives to maintain a healthy pH balance of between 7.3 and 7.4 to protect our cells from getting burned and destroyed by these acids. But there are times when it can no longer achieve this.

When acidity levels in the body exceed a certain threshold, the person is described as being "hyperacidified". They feel listless, exhausted, worn out and overwhelmed by everyday life. It may also be the cause of several chronic diseases.

When this happens, the body is forced to bind the excess acid to its stock of mineral salts, to neutralize it and store it as waste product.

What can be done about this? An intake of mineral salts can restore the balance but unfortunately, our modern diet often doesn't contain sufficient amounts of mineral salts to keep you healthy.

Linus Pauling, the Nobel prize-winning chemist said: *"Every disease is directly linked to a lack of mineral salts"*. This being the case, two thirds of the food we eat should contain mineral salts.

Each mineral salt plays an essential role in your body. In the case of hyperacidity, like plants, the human body tries to procure alkalizers, such as calcium for example. But, and this is the most worrying thing, if there's a lack of calcium in your diet, your body dips into its reserves (from your bones, for example)! The result is severe demineralization that gets worse as time goes on.

And you get sick.

Researchers have discovered that there are more than two hundred degenerative diseases which are directly linked to a lack of calcium; diseases such as diabetes, joint disease (arthritis, arthrosis and rheumatism), heart disease, kidney stones, gallstones and cancer. Cancer, according to specialists, is often nothing more than the result of a catastrophic hyper-acidification of the body over decades.

The human body – a walking garbage dump?

The connective tissue, bloodstream, lungs and kidneys work continuously to rid the body of harmful acidic waste.

Connective tissue is just as important as blood. It performs a regulatory function that every organ in our body depends on. It's essentially a fertile source of nourishment for the cells. Just as a plant depends on the quality of the earth in which it grows, human cells depend on the quality of the connective tissue. If you exercise and consume enough mineral salts, your connective tissue will usually be able to eliminate accumulated waste product. But if it reaches the point where it can no longer do this, the result is the release of a catastrophic surplus of acid, the most minor signs of which are, for example, heartburn.

What happens when acids reach a saturation point in the body?

Put simply, connective tissue is a massive warehouse for waste product. When the kidneys can no longer eliminate acidic waste, this toxic waste accumulates in the connective tissue.

This means the toxins are stored, for example in your joints, when they shouldn't be. Doctors who specialize in hyperacidity say that arthrosis, rheumatism and polyarthritis are triggered by the built up deposits of surplus acid and other biological toxins in the body.

This is very serious because, in the long term, excess acidity in the body is synonymous with disease. To spell it out; acid gradually undermines the functioning of our bodies in different ways, ultimately ruining our health completely.

Let's do a simple test:

Let's take two apples, spraying only one with a coral water solution (coral water is rich in coral minerals and has a high calcium content).

After three months, a clear difference can be seen: the apple sprayed with coral water looks almost as fresh as the day it was picked, while the other apple is withered and wrinkled.

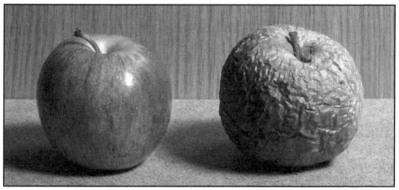

The apple on the left has been sprayed with a coral water solution while the one on the right has not. Both apples were then left for three months.

What does this mean?

It shows that the aging of an organism depends, to an extent, on the state of its connective tissue. The cells and organic systems of connective tissue saturated with acids will age faster. But when an organism – in our case the apple, is sprayed with a coral water solution, it's protected and gets enough calcium to stay healthy. The same is true for the human body.

It's simple: taking in more calcium gives you greater protection against excess acidity and therefore ensures much better health.

It has now been proven that almost all diseases, particularly chronic ones, are linked to a dysfunction of the body's pH-balance.

Calcium and cancer

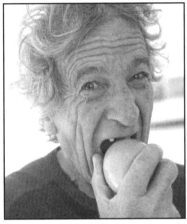

Today, we know that there's a direct link between calcium deficiency and disease. Could a similar correlation exist between calcium deficiency and cancer?

Carcinogens are highly reactive free radicals. They infiltrate your body through the food you eat and the air your breathe. For example, saturated fatty acid, food additives such as nitrates, inhaling the benzol and tar in cigarettes, and even second-hand smoke are ways in which your body can be infiltrated.

Your body has various defence mechanisms for protecting its cells against the attack of these carcinogens. In a healthy cellular liquid with a sufficient supply of calcium and an acceptable pH value between 7.4 and 6.6, these mutated receptors (free radicals) cannot form.

This means that a healthy, slightly alkaline, cellular environment, with sufficient calcium levels, is not an environment in which a cancer could grow. The calcium factor could then play a determining role in the future treatment of cancer.

Calcium and heart disease

Heart disease is the number one killer in the US and Europe where one in two will die of a heart-related disease (and one in three will die from cancer). The catastrophic and often fatal hyperacidity infiltrates the cardiac muscle after years of excess acid in the body. The principal aspect of heart disease is not the biochemical function of the cardiac muscle, but rather, the composition of the liquid that feeds the muscle, in other words the blood!

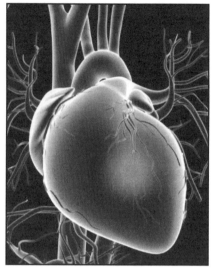

New research has shown that the ability of the heart muscle to contract and relax depends on the ionization of calcium. Deposits (plaques) form in the arteries, thickening and hardening their walls (arteriosclerosis). These deposits can be attributed to different causes, but most of all to a lack of exercise and poor diet.

If excess acid accumulates in this environment, it attacks and destroys the muscular layer of the arteries. This triggers a defence mechanism in the body, which tries to seal the damaged muscular layers with the deposits to "plug up" the holes. If it didn't do this, the arteries could tear, causing instant death.

But if the level of calcium ions was high enough to maintain the ideal pH balance at 7.4, the deterioration of the cells caused by the excess acidity in the organic liquids would never even occur. The body wouldn't need to make these repairs.

Calcium and osteoporosis

Likewise, for women, hormonal deficiencies play a fundamental role. The production of estrogen, the feminine hormone that performs an essential regulatory function in the bones, slows with the onset of menopause and becomes imbalanced.

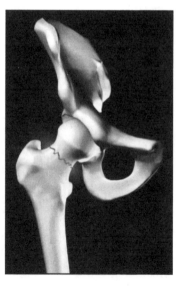

At this point, parathormone (which is responsible for maintaining the calcium levels in the bloodstream at a precise level, simultaneously protecting against the deterioration of the bones) comes into play.

This is particularly serious when your diet is not sufficiently rich in calcium, or when excess acid means the body is forced to use up its inventory of calcium to balance out these acids.

Remember: your body needs calcium, and if it doesn't get enough through the food you eat, it ransacks its own reserves. In other words: to maintain the pH of the blood as close as possible to 7.4, the body draws the calcium it needs from the bones. The result is a pathological decalcification of the bones (osteoporosis) that occurs when a mineral salt deficiency makes the bones increasingly fragile. So, brittle bones have more to do with a lack of calcium than with growing old!

Calcium and arthrosis, arthritis and rheumatic diseases

Did you know that epicondylitis (tennis elbow) and bursitis are the first signs of catastrophic levels of excess acid in the body?

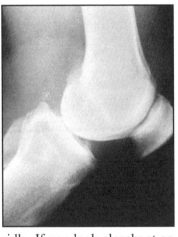

There's no doubt that excess acid in the body is one of the causes of cartilage death. Basically, chronic calcium deficiency along with the surplus acid this causes, alters the synovial fluid (the liquid which lubricates the joints) and which also serves to nourish the cartilage. The cartilage doesn't get the nutrients it needs and so it begins to deteriorate rapidly. If you look closely at an x-ray of an elbow with epicondylitis, you can clearly see that the arthritic joints are pitted with holes where they have been attacked by acid.

Artrosis, arthritis and rheumatic pain is the result of excess acid attacking the joints, tendons, muscles, bursae and nerves. A body suffering from excess acidity, having saturated the connective tissue with acidic waste, will store this same waste in the tendons, muscles, nervous system and joints.

Calcium and digestion problems

Calcium deficiency and excess acid also have an impact on your digestion. When your liver, gall bladder and pancreas cannot produce enough alkaline substances to neutralize the acid chyme in the stomach, foods that have not been properly digested are channelled towards deeper sections of the intestine. The change in the bacterial climate paralyzes intestinal activity and as a result, the body does not get enough of the nutrients and mineral salts it needs.

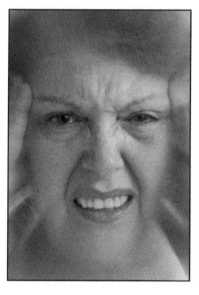

Calcium and fatigue, low energy levels and concentration problems

If your metabolic system is acidic and deprived of sufficient calcium, your energy levels plummet and you'll sleep badly. Your over-acidified body begins to secrete more stress hormones. And in the constant battle to overcome the excess acid, your body becomes exhausted. But, when the presence of calcium ions in the body is sufficient, you feel better, more invigorated and you sleep better.

Calcium and back and/or disc problems

Excess acidity makes the muscles rigid. They tense up and may also block the nerves which can cause aches and pains. In the case of a disc hernia, a part of the disc, which has lost its elasticity, protrudes between two vertebra in the spinal column and gets jammed in between them, potentially pinching certain nerve endings. The loss of elasticity of the disc, which is made up primarily of collagen, is also often due to the aging of the collagen tissue caused by the acids. The protective sheath covering the nerves is made up of connective tissue, which is also used as a store for acid! The acid irritates the nerves, which in turn causes pain.

Inflammatory disease: What is it?

Now that you have a general understanding of inflammatory disease, you can see why it's called "inflammatory". You're now going to discover how you can efficiently fight these conditions. The inflammatory diseases you're now going to read about are:

- Heart attacks
- Diabetes
- Arthrosis, arthritis and rheumatism
- Cardiovascular disease
- Crohn's disease
- Strokes
- Cancer
- Alzheimer's disease

You are going to discover a completely new way of looking at these types of diseases... and in doing so you're going to be half way towards solving the problem (because you'll have identified the cause of these diseases). This is going to give you a good chance of seeing them from all angles and doing so is going to allow you to find new, efficient ways of curing them.

Inflammatory diseases and their causes

Imagine that you're walking through a forest when, on the ground by the side of the path, you notice some branches glowing faintly and giving off smoke. You know it hasn't rained for several days and so your first thought is that the glowing embers could be the start of a fire that could end up engulfing the whole forest.

What would you do? That's easy: You'd stamp out these first few flames, so it didn't get any worse.

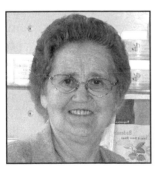

Jeannette L., 68 years old, of R. (Ref. 7304)

"The end of my back pain and headaches!"

"Ever since I was a child I've suffered dreadful headaches, accompanied by a burning sensation in the nape of my neck and back. When I woke up in the night, in particular, the pain would start in the back of my head and spread outwards to my back. Physicians couldn't work out what was causing it and were unable to help me.

Last January 7, my life changed. I woke up and wasn't in any pain at all. What had happened? It was definitely due to the Antarctic Krill Oil with Coral Calcium I had started taking five days prior. My pharmacist recommended it, but I never imagined it would work so well and so fast."

15

Your body "burns"...

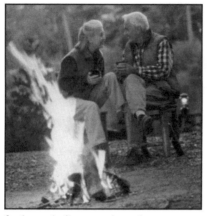

Let's transfer this example to your body. When you cut yourself, you first clean the wound to kill any germs to keep it from getting infected. You do this because you know that if you don't, you're risking a painful inflammation or even serious blood poisoning. It's the logical thing to do.

But what do you do if you feel an inflammation, but you can't even see it? From the pain, you know there's a problem, but you don't know exactly where the pain is coming from. In other words: you're suffering from chronic pain but you ignore the fact that it's being caused by an inflammation.

But just like a cut, if you don't do anything to treat it, this "internal" inflammation will grow and grow. Your body is "on fire", yet you don't know what to do about it. Recent medical studies even speak of a phenomenon called "inflammatory stress"!

Internal and external inflammation

So, as there are inflammations and infected swellings that you can easily see (and treat) on the outside of your body, there are also inflammations that you CANNOT see inside your body!

It's only been recently discovered that heart attacks, insulin resistance, strokes, diabetes, Alzheimer's and cancer are closely linked to inflammatory processes inside the body. So, it should make sense to treat these diseases as inflammations, since this is exactly what our bodies do.

The body does have a mechanism to combat inflammation, but once this defensive process has been triggered, it doesn't stop. The body never halts this process which it itself launches. The center of the inflammation spreads onwards and outwards.

How ordinary inflammatory diseases can trigger a heart attack or stroke

Heart attacks and strokes aren't just caused by the clogging up of the blood vessels with fatty deposits. Recent research points to the first changes in the vessels starting in early life, around the age of fifteen.

Risk factors

The risk factors promoting the obstruction of the blood vessels, thus making the much-feared heart attack more likely, are:

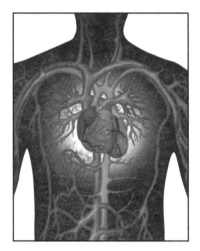

- **Family history (genetic predisposition)**
- **Excess weight and obesity**
- **Smoking**
- **Lack of physical exercise**
- **Age   – Stress**
- **Excess fatty deposits in the bloodstream (cholesterol, triglycerides)**
- **High blood pressure**
- **Sugar and diabetes**
- **Gender (male, female)**
- **Arteriosclerosis**

Of course, these aren't the only causes of death due to cardiovascular disease. But there's no doubt that these are all factors that are harmful to your cardiovascular system. By knowing this, you should learn to change the way you think and find out more about the subject.

Traditional risk factors are not the cause

Did you know that half of all heart attacks happen to people with normal cholesterol levels? In two thirds of all heart attacks and strokes, the blood vessels were not found to be constricted, or were only slightly constricted. Likewise, there are many people who are in good health despite having high cholesterol levels. It has also been proven that a heart by-pass operation, which should restore good circulation in our bloodstream, does not definitely prevent further heart attacks. People who are not overweight, who don't smoke, who don't have unusually high fatty deposits in their blood and who have normal blood pressure can also die of a heart attack.

So, you need to look beyond the "traditional" risk factors. As we suspected, inflammatory reaction plays an essential role. To help us understand it better, we need to look further into the cholesterol issue, so often referred to in the case of inflammatory disease, but first, let's clear up one major misunderstanding about cholesterol...

Cholesterol

The bottom line is, cholesterol is NOT to be feared or fought! Why?

Cholesterol is vital

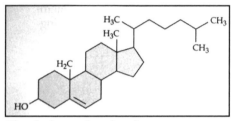

The cholesterol molecule

Cholesterol performs an important function in your body. It gives the cell walls their stability and elasticity and plays a role in the production of a series of hormones. Your body needs cholesterol for the production of vitamin D as a raw material in your brain and nerve cells. Bile acid, which your body needs to burn fats, is made from cholesterol. Nature gives you sufficient quantities of cholesterol; your body absorbs nearly 0.5 grams of it every day through your diet. And your body even produces its own cholesterol; around 1 gram a day, specifically in the liver and in the small intestine.

For a balanced body: An egg for breakfast, with some butter!

Here's an interesting phenomenon: when you banish fats from your diet, your body produces more cholesterol. If, on the other hand, you eat a hyperlipidic diet (very rich in fats), the body halts its cholesterol production. Your body is constantly striving to maintain a balance. You may not always be aware of it, but inevitably the consequences are going to make themselves felt. By giving up your daily egg and not putting any butter on your bread, you're only reducing your cholesterol levels by 3%. As well as cholesterol, your blood also contains triglycerides (neutral fats), which you absorb through your diet or from the supply of carbohydrates that your body stores as an energy reserve.

An imbalance with some very heavy consequences

There are primitive tribes, such as the Masai, who eat twice the amount of fats we do, yet they suffer a far lower rate of cardiovascular disease. Within Europe, there are population groups with a very high risk of cardiovascular disease and others with a low risk. For example, the French and the Spanish eat as much fat as the Germans, yet they have a much lower rate of heart attacks and strokes. From this, we can conclude that the quantity of fats absorbed is not a determining factor in the risk of being struck by a cardiovascular disease. What is a determining factor, however, is the type and quality of fat consumed. Basically, as you may perhaps already know, not all fats are the same.

Fat burners are anti-inflammatories

An interesting large-scale study carried out at Harvard University on approximately 80,000 women, showed that taking existing anti-cholesterol medication made only a very small contribution to limiting heart attacks and strokes.

Only the introduction of new agents, such as statins or fat burners, gave any significant reduction in risk levels. It seems that cholesterol reducers stabilize the vessel walls, enabling them to fight existing or imminent inflammation. These new medicines have one thing in common: they are anti-inflammatories.

This means that, in the correct formulation, this medicine designed initially to protect the vessel walls and reduce cholesterol also has another

---

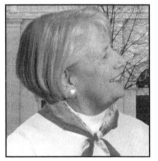

Mary H., 63 years old, of S. (Ref. 5661)

"Finally free of my joint pain!"

"Every time I knelt in church to pray and then got up again, the pain in my joints was terrible. It finally got to the point where I just couldn't kneel. You can't possibly understand what that meant to me!

My pharmacist insisted I try Antarctic Krill Oil with Coral Calcium, 100% biologically assimilable. And it worked! Exactly ten days later, my pain was much less. I now feel ten years younger.

I got my life back. I feel happy again, I can laugh and enjoy myself. And best of all, I can work normally once more, out in the fresh air, in the garden I love so much."

effect: "encircling the heart of the fire" and confining the inflammation.

This is going to serve to protect against both heart attacks and strokes alike.

Free radicals feed the heart of the fire

There is a difference between "good" and "bad" cholesterol, in other words, HDL cholesterol and LDL cholesterol. The first one, HDL ("good cholesterol") is useful, essential even. It gathers the cholesterol present in the blood and transports it to the liver. The other, LDL cholesterol, ("bad cholesterol") plays a role in the formation of plaques, in other words, fatty deposits on the artery walls. The liver cells are responsible for identifying and eliminating cholesterol. But once the LDL cholesterol has been oxidized, the liver cells can no longer detect them.

Where does the oxidized cholesterol come from?

You have certainly heard about free radicals. They cause oxidation. But do you know what exactly are free radicals and their effect on your body?

Free radicals easily explained

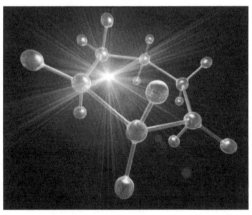

A free radical is an atom or a molecule with at least one unpaired electron and which will try to statiblize itself by "stealing" an electron from a nearby molecule thereby causing oxidative cell damage.

Some free radicals appear normally during metabolism. Sometimes the body's immune system's cells creates them on purpose to neutralize viruses and bacteria. However, environmental factors such as pollution, radiation, cigarette smoke and herbicides can also spawn free radicals.

Free radicals are very unstable and react quickly with other compounds, trying to capture the needed electron to gain stability. Generally, free radicals attack the nearest stable molecule, "stealing" its electron.

When the "attacked" molecule loses its electron, it becomes a free radical itself, beginning a chain reaction. Once the process is started, it can cascade, finally resulting in the disruption of a living cell.

The destructive power of free radicals and oxidative stress

Normally, the body can handle free radicals, but if antioxidants are unavailable, or if the free radical production becomes excessive, damage can occur. The oxidative chain reaction causes inflammation and makes the cells age. It can also cause alterations in the cells that make them more susceptible to different types of cancers. Of particular importance is that free radical damage accumulates with age.

Free radicals interact with other molecules within cells. This can cause oxidative damage (stress) to proteins, membranes and genes. Oxidative damage has been implicated in the cause of many diseases and has an impact on the aging process. Examples of such diseases are:

– **Heart attacks**	– **Parkinson's disease**
– **Cataracts**	– **Arthrosis, arthritis and rheumatism**
– **Cancer**	– **Alzheimer's disease**

Oxidative stress can be aggravated when the metabolic environment is complicated by:

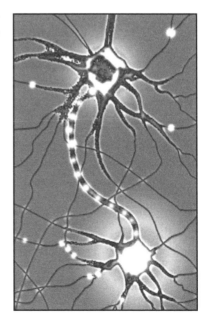

- **Alcohol consumption**
- **Sugar and diabetes**
- **Inflammations**
- **Infections**
- **Some medicines**
- **The ozone and UV rays**
- **X-rays**
- **Stress and smoking**
- **Excess weight and obesity**
- **Contaminants such as air pollution and pesticides.**

21

Inflammation of the blood vessels

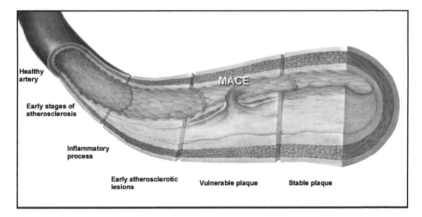

Inflammed blood vessel

For a long time it was believed that the deterioration of the blood vessel walls resulted from a mechanical stimulus. Under the influence of blood fats, residues containing cholesterol were deposited on the inside of the arterial blood vessels, which could lead to a heart attack. These deposits, known as plaques, "stick" to the artery walls. It was always assumed that these plaques got bigger, obstructing the circulation of the blood, resulting in restricted blood flow which could then lead to either a heart attack or a stroke.

Heart attacks and strokes

According to recent research, atherosclerosis-related heart attacks and strokes (where the vessels become altered) are actually caused by an inflammatory process. Here, chronic inflammatory reactions bring about changes to the blood vessels, causing a reaction comparable to an inflammation of the skin that degenerates into a burn.

Inflammation sites in your body

The exact process has not yet fully emerged and is still under research, but more and more signs point to the existence of pockets of inflammation inside the body that, over the course of time, gradually block the blood vessels, spreading and propagating ever outwards.

In other words:

Contrary to the theory of the obstruction of the arteries, *the real cause of heart attacks and strokes is, in all likelihood, an inflammation in the blood vessels and corresponding organs.*

Destroying fats encourages inflammation

Oxidized fats are the body's alarm bell. When fats such as oxidized LDL (bad) cholesterol are floating in the bloodstream, the liver has no way to see or eliminate them. The immune system, however, identifies them as foreign bodies and summons immune-system cells, also called "scavenger cells" or macrophages, which have one sole objective: destroy intruders (which is what the oxidized fats are).

The inflammatory activity boost

These immune-system cells that cause inflammation then burrow into the artery wall and begin gobbling up droplets of fat. These fat-filled cells form a plaque and inflammation thins its fibrous cap. Eventually, the cap ruptures, and the plaque's contents spill into the bloodstream – along with pro-inflammatory cytokines, which encourage clotting. Suddenly, the artery fills with a cloud of rapidly coagulating blood cells. If the cloud is large enough, it forms a clot that blocks the artery and causes a heart attack or stroke.

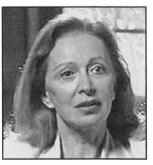

Solange C., 48 years old, of P. (Ref. 984)

"My chronic osteoporosis eased and the aches and pains have disappeared!"

"I've suffered from serious osteoporosis and osteoarthritis. I'd also developed nodules on my fingers and feet and the base of my spine. Just a few months after I started taking Antarctic Krill Oil with Coral Calcium, they disappeared.

All my aches and pains have also disappeared. And my osteoporosis, which was quite advanced, is steadily improving. In any event, thanks to Antarctic Krill Oil and a little exercise, I've really been feeling very well!"

Oxidized fats

The more of these there are, the more harmful inflammation-boosting substances are secreted. This may happen gradually over the course of decades. That's why older people are more vulnerable to death by heart attack than the young.

How can we prevent inflammatory diseases inside our body?

The best way to prevent, and even halt the progress, of inflammatory disease in our body is to take substances with anti-inflammatory properties. When the body is healthy, it can get everything it needs from food and absorb it properly. But when the body is weakened and sick, as a result of a poor diet or because of pollution or a lack of exercise, it just doesn't have the capacity to do this. That's why for many years now, we've all been keeping an eye on our fat intake; choosing vegetable oil, preferably sunflower, safflower, sweet corn oil or, best of all, olive oil, as well as products made with these oils, over animal fats such as butter.

Omega-6 and Omega-3 fatty acids

But what you probably haven't known for all these years, is that these oils have a high content of Omega-6 fatty acids. Of course, overall they contain less saturated (bad) fats, but did you know that there is an imbalance between the Omega-6 and Omega-3 fatty acids in the polyunsaturated (good) fats they contain?

You need Omega-3 fatty acids to control the inflammatory process inside our body. We'll come back to this point later on. For now, just remember that a misunderstanding like this can cause damage to our blood vessels since it increases the risk of constriction and coagulation. So what can you do? Make sure that you get enough Omega-3!

How can you increase your Omega-3 intake?

One way of increasing your Omega-3 intake is by eating more fish. It contains Omega-3 EPA (eicosapentaenoic acid) and DHA (docosahexaenoic acid). So, fish is very healthy. However, not all fish are equally rich in Omega-3.

Cold water fish and Omega-3

Coldwater fish such as mackerel, salmon, herring, tuna and sardines, which eat plankton, contain high levels of Omega-3 EPA and DHA. The colder the water they live in, the richer they are in Omega-3 fatty acids which keep the cellular envelopes of the fish "liquid". This ensures they remain mobile and can survive in the glacial waters of, for example, the Antarctic Ocean (whereas, trout and carp, who live in warmer waters, contain far lower levels of Omega-3).

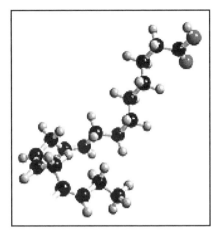

The Omega-3 molecule

Krill's special Omega-3 content

Krill contains particularly powerful Omega-3 fatty acids which are extremely effective because they're linked to phospholipids, a chemical structure that increases their bioavailability (in other words, the body absorbs them better). This is not true of ordinary fish oils, in which Omega-3 is linked to triglycerides.

The pages which follow contains a wealth of information on the valuable Omega-3 properties of Krill.

Fish on the menu!

Generally, fish makes up a fairly small part of our diet, so our Omega-3 intake is seriously lacking. It's recommended that we eat two portions of fish per week, yet only 21% of the American population ever eats fish, while in other countries, the average intake is only around a half portion per week.

The vast majority of us aren't getting enough Omega-3! In other words, we are suffering from an Omega-3 deficiency.

Fish oil capsules: A Godsend?

Even if there's no fish on the menu, we still need to get our recommended dose of Omega-3! So, why not simply take fish oil capsules that contain high concentrations of easily absorbed Omega-3?

Of course, some vegetable oils such as linseed oil, canola oil and walnut oil – also contain Omega-3. But they contain the short-chain variety that needs to be converted into the long-chain type before it can have the positive effect on the vessels described below. You would need to consume huge quantities of these oils (and calories) to obtain the same benefits you get from a very small quantity of long-chain fatty acids found in coldwater fish.

Find out what some native people know about staying healthy

Let's take a flight over our blue planet and pause for a moment to zoom in on the native people of Greenland, the Inuit (previously called the Eskimos). They rarely suffer from high blood pressure, cholesterol problems or inflammatory disease of joints or skin, and heart attacks are a very infrequent occurrence. We think it's because they eat a lot of fish. But, that's not the whole story.

According to the research available on the subject, the fats in fish possess innumerable vasoprotective properties (i.e. they protect the blood vessels) making them an absolutely unique resource. They have a beneficial action on the way fats are metabolized and can reduce the high triglyceride levels common in diabetics. They also bring down "bad cholesterol" while at the same time increasing "good cholesterol".

These fatty acids help to normalize high blood pressure and promote blood irrigation. They increase the elasticity of the red blood cells, making them circulate more easily through the narrow blood vessels. The blood stays liquid, facilitating the delivery of oxygen and nutrients to the tiniest blood vessels. What's more, these fatty acids prevent the clumping together of the red blood cells, which is vital for optimal blood flow.

Omega-3 EPA and DHA normalize heart arrhythmia and can provide protection against a sudden heart attack. They combat and halt harmful inflammatory processes in the vessels, joints, digestive system, skin and other parts of the body.

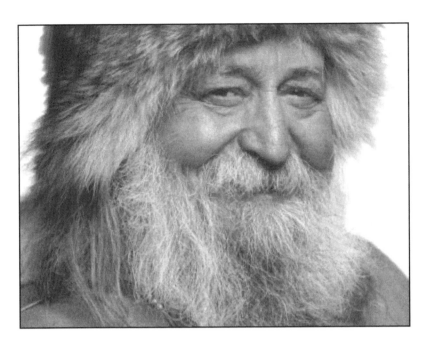

Here's what and how Omega-3 protects

In short: Omega-3 (EPA and DHA, found in fish and fish oil) is

---

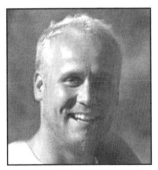

Mr. John R., of O. (Ref: 12360)

"My doctor couldn't believe my cholesterol level!"

"I can't tell you how much I like Antarctic Krill Oil. My treatment has made my hair silkier. My skin is softer and people tell me I look radiant. Before, I used to burn quickly in the sun and never really got a tan. Now I can be out in the sun for hours, without any sunscreen, and I never get sunburned – it's amazing! I can also attest that my cholesterol level is down so much, that my doctor was stunned. He'd never seen results like it! I've trusted natural medicines for years, but this product is the best I've ever tried and I'd recommend it to anybody."

a natural substance with many different benefits that can be used effectively in cases of:

High blood pressure: – they boost blood irrigation

Inflammation: – they increase blood flow

Heart arrhythmia: – they promote good cholesterol (HDL)
   – they aid the synthesis of triglycerides
   – they combat blood clotting

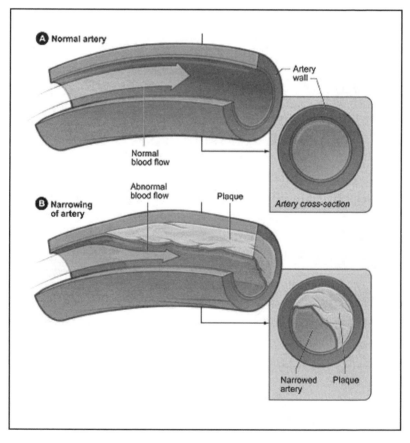

Healthy artery (top) and the gradually narrowing of the artery caused by fatty deposits and cholesterol (bottom).

How to protect yourself against heart attacks and strokes

The Japanese, like the Inuit have a much lower mortality rate from heart attacks than we do in the West. On the Japanese island of Okinawa, where fish consumption is at a level almost double that found on the main islands of the Japanese archipelago, which is itself three times higher than in the USA... the incidence of heart attacks is even lower than that on the mainland and much, much lower than in the USA.

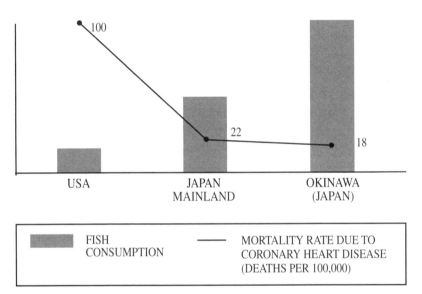

	FISH CONSUMPTION	MORTALITY RATE DUE TO CORONARY HEART DISEASE (DEATHS PER 100,000)

SOURCES: World Health Organization, 1996; Japan Ministry of Health and Welfare; Clinical laboratory medecine, 2nd Edition, Kenneth D. McClatchey (et al.), Food and Agriculture Organization of the United Nations (FAO).

Lots of fish: yes, but...

A study published in 2004 shows that people who have a regular intake of Omega-3 have a lower risk of suffering a stroke. Just eating fish two to four times per week brings the risk down by 20%! Eating coldwater fish (at least five times per week) brings your stroke risk down by up to 30%!!

Unfortunately, for many of us, eating fish in these quantities on a regular basis throughout our lives is difficult, which is why it's common to take supplements in capsules or in soft gel capsules.

Omega-3 in soft gel capsules

Taking Omega-3 in a soft gel capsule form is a way to ensure that we get our recommended intake of Omega-3, but very few of us take advantage of this. But now, to protect you against the two biggest killers of our time, inflammatory disease and hyperacidity, there finally exists a new generation of capsules: the new Antarctic Krill Oil soft gel capsules!

Antarctic Krill – the new generation of Omega-3

Comparative studies have shown that Antarctic Krill Oil soft gel capsules are vastly more effective than regular fish oil capsules. Antarctic Krill Oil contains 48 times more antioxidants than regular Omega-3 fish oil (yes, 48 times more!). It's better tolerated and can be used for a wider variety of treatments, because it combats both inflammation and excess acidity (thanks to its unique combination of Omega-3 and calcium). What's more, Antarctic Krill Oil soft gel capsules have no unpleasant side effects, such as belching (fishy-smelling burps).

The Omega-3 in Antarctic Krill Oil is linked to phospholipids, constituents of lecithin and human cell membranes. This is the reason why the body absorbs them more easily than the triglycerides in fish oil. Antarctic Krill Oil is easily digestible and lighter than any vegetable source of Omega-3 such as linseed, hemp, canola and walnut oils. Despite their undeniable health benefits, these oils require bile acid for their assimilation, meaning that only a tiny proportion can be transformed into a truly valuable active ingredient.

There are also many people who find it difficult to digest fats. For these people, Antarctic Krill Oil now certainly provides the safest and best-tolerated way of taking Omega-3. Only one or two soft gel capsules per day of Antarctic Krill Oil is sufficient to quickly observe its many amazing health benefits. Its ease of absorption and infinitely superior properties are undoubtedly the reason why Antarctic Krill Oil beats fish oil hands-down in every comparative study.

Antarctic Krill Oil stands out for its unique combination of anti-oxidants from astaxanthin, vitamins A and E as well as rare flavonoids, giving it its amazing anti-oxidant capacity of 378 units/g. That's nearly 300 times the capacity of vitamins A and E and nearly 50 times greater than fish, endowing Antarctic Krill Oil with its notable stability and keeping it free of any rancid taste – another advantage it has over fish oil, linseed oil and other sources of Omega-3 which, if oxidized, can even be harmful.

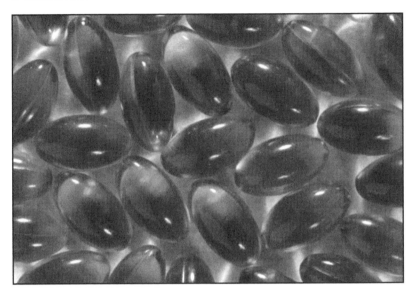

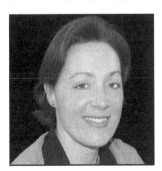

Mrs. Louise M., 46 years old, of H. (Ref: 20174)

"My general state of health is much improved ."

"I've been taking Antarctic Krill Oil soft gel capsules for a month now, and everything written about it in the press is true. I could hardly move and suffered terrible pain, but everything improved in a very short space of time. It wasn't long ago that I couldn't even put any weight on my right leg. Now it's not a problem. The pain in my elbow, caused by a fall, is almost gone. Since I've been taking Antarctic Krill Oil, my general state of health, both physical and mental is much improved. I'm going to carry on taking it and would strongly recommend it to anyone."

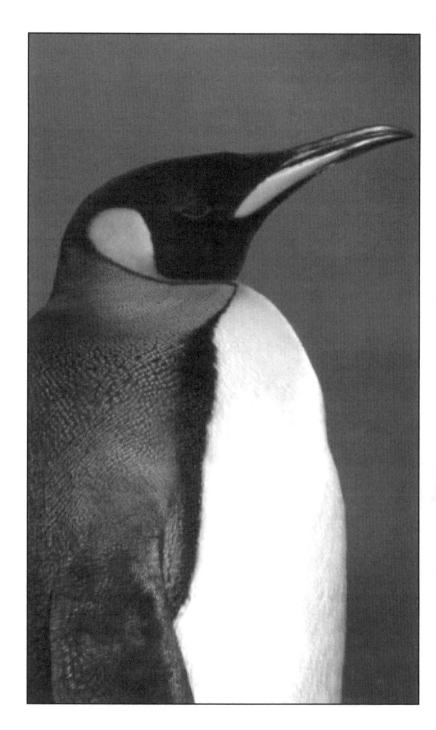

CHAPTER 2
Why don't penguins have cholesterol problems despite their extremely fatty diet?

The cure that came in from the cold – Mother Nature's perfect food: Antarctic Krill

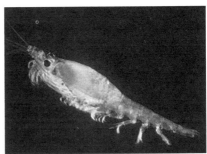

From the clear blue, glacial waters of the Antarctic comes an oil so powerful it can radically change your life. Krill oil improves your health, fortifies your immune system and can even cure chronic disease.

Do you know why penguins don't suffer from cholesterol problems, despite eating a diet incredibly rich in fat?

The answer is simple: It's because they eat Krill !

Based at the Artiga research station in the Antarctic since 1995, Doctor Grillo has been studying the effects of Krill on the animal organism. He noticed that no penguins, regardless of age, had any kind of arteriosclerotic deposits in their blood vessels despite eating such an incredibly fatty diet! He concluded that it was as a result of their diet, comprised essentially of Krill.

Could it be that the diet of the Antarctic penguin is hiding the solution to hyperacidity, inflammatory diseases, joint diseases, cholesterol problems, heart attacks, strokes and even cancers, all of which are among the greatest scourges of our times?

What is Krill?

Krill is a Norwegian word meaning "whale food". It's the generic name for the tiny crustaceans that live in large schools. They form the basis of the Antarctic ecosystem and provide the principle source of food for whales, seals, icefish, cuttlefish, penguins and albatrosses. Of the 85 known species, the most commonly found

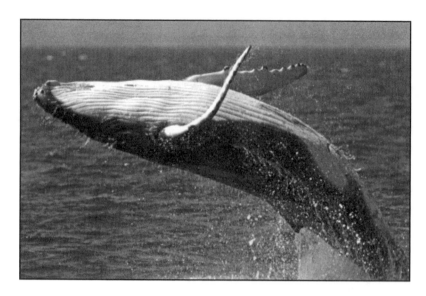

is *Euphausia superba*, also called "Antarctic Krill". It exists in such enormous quantities that we could cover the complete surface area of the USA (4 million square miles) three and a half times over with 1,700 tons of Krill per square mile!

The Antarctic Ocean harbors up to 6.7 billion tons of Krill, with potential human consumption of between only 50 and 150 million tons per year. Krill reproduces very rapidly and doesn't have any natural predators to worry about, so its survival is assured, guaranteeing mankind access to its benefits for centuries to come.

The results of laboratory tests show that Krill is also effective at preventing and combating diseases caused by the build-up of fatty deposits in the blood vessels.

Since the beginning of the nineties, Krill "meat" has been available in some supermarkets. But few people know about Krill or its health benefits.

Krill exists in abundance

It contains one of the most powerful combinations of antioxidants and nutrients. There is every chance of it becoming one of the major foodstuffs in our future. Hardly a day goes by without another study somewhere in the world confirming the therapeutic and nutritional benefits of Krill oil.

It all starts with Krill!

Krill is right at the bottom of the food chain. It feeds on vegetable plankton and is therefore, unpolluted by the heavy metals and pesticides that contaminate most fish.

In the production of the oil, Krill is only harvested in tiny quantities, so as not to disturb the environment and to preserve the delicate balance of the food chain.

Krill feed on algae *(diatomaceous)* and phytoplankton, which accumulates and enters the composition of the oil procured from these tiny crustaceans.

Krill Oil contains:

– **Krill-based Omega-3 anti-inflammatories**
– **Phospholipids that protect and stimulate the brain**
– **Antioxidants that protect the cells**

We've given a name to this oil:

Antarctic Krill Oil

Antarctic Krill Oil contains the three high-performance nutrients listed above (Omega-3, phospholipids and powerful antioxidants) in significant quantities.

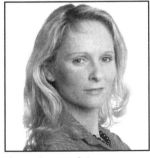

Mrs. Ursula A., of B., therapist
(Ref: 20174)

"Antarctic Krill gives off good energy, I've adopted it!"

"I'm an independent therapist and I've been taking Antarctic Krill (with Coral Calcium) since 2007 (and my husband takes it too). I think it's an excellent product. I tested it on my patients using bioresonance therapy and the results were largely very positive. Antarctic Krill Oil really is an effective treatment for chronic inflammation and arthrosis. It reduces the symptoms in patients with chronic hyperacidity. Antarctic Krill Oil gives off good energy, I've adopted it!"

According to specialists, these substances endow Antarctic Krill with the power to resolve even the most extreme health issues. Each component makes its own special contribution, and together they work in synergy to efficiently combat many health issues such as, for example, premenstrual syndrome (cramps, mood swings), hypercholesterolemia and joint pain (arthrosis, arthritis, rheumatism, etc...) to name only a few.

The ingredients of Antarctic Krill Oil contain everything you need to confront the stresses and strains of our modern lives.

Antioxidants

Antioxidants neutralize free radicals. They are an essential component of breast milk. They help the baby build its defences against infection. They're found in garlic, ginger, linseed, brown rice, berries, rosemary and basil.

Krill and antioxidants

Tests have shown that Antarctic Krill Oil contains an impressive cocktail of powerful antioxidants. In addition to the general health benefits, this also makes this oil very stable (for example, these antioxidants don't have the fishy aftertaste of other Omega-3 oils). And, these antioxidants (like Astaxanthin) are stellar active anti-aging ingredients. In other words, in sufficient quantities, Antarctic Krill Oil, can slow the aging process!

One of the features of astaxanthin is that it's fully esterified,

The Astaxanthin powerfull anti-aging anti-oxidant molecule found in Krill Oil.

which means it's linked to the EPA and DHA molecules, which are derivatives of the cellular metabolism of the Krill. This means the body can absorb it completely, maximizing all its extraordinary antioxidant properties. Also, the astaxanthin can cross the blood-brain barrier, which protects and stimulates the brain.

A new flavonoid

Antarctic Krill also contains a new flavonoid which scientists have named *Sampalis*. This substance, usually found in plants, has remarkable antioxidant properties.

On the ORAC scale (Oxygen Radical Absorbance Capacity), Antarctic Krill has record high antioxidant capacity score!

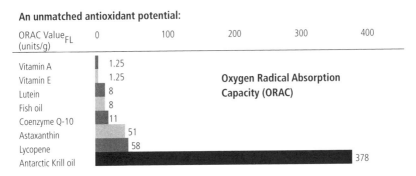

In direct comparison with other known antioxidants available in the form of oils as mentioned above, Antarctic Krill scored an amazing 378. This is 300 times higher than vitamins A and E, which are powerful antioxidants in their own right, and 48 times higher than the antioxidant capacity of standard Omega-3 fish oils.

These days, the health benefits of Omega-3 fatty acids are widely accepted. They constitute vital elements of the cellular membrane and are essential for the proper functioning of the central nervous system. They play an eminent role in the regulation of clotting, blood pressure and inflammation. But dieticians tell us our diet contains a proportion of Omega-6 fatty acids (found primarily in cereal and vegetables oils, meat, poultry and eggs) which is too high (between 10 and 20 times too high). It is only by remedying this imbalance that the body will be able to manage its fatty acids.

So, our body needs Omega-3 just as much as it needs Omega-6. Both are essential for blocking the inflammation process. But the excess Omega-6 that we consume upsets the balance.

Antarctic Krill Oil has the potential to re-establish the balance, because the Krill Oil content makes it extremely rich in Omega-3.

Finally: phospholipids

Every single cell in our body needs phospholipids: they enter the composition of the cell membranes. Also called "cell sentinels", they form a microscopic barrier that allows the cell to filter out the toxins that cause disease.

The phospholipidic content of red blood cells is 45%. Your brain also contains a high proportion of phospholipids. They accelerate the cellular metabolism and ensure vital elements penetrate the cell while at the same time evacuating any unwanted ones. Phospholipids also nourish the skin.

An interesting feature of the phospholipids in Antarctic Krill Oil is that they resemble the ones found in the human brain, which is the part of the body where the cellular membrane is richest in phospholipids.

Now let's put these powerful, essential substances together!

Putting these substances together makes a highly effective product that prevents and cures disease, and boosts regeneration processes! A product that's 100% natural and contains nothing but the very best ingredients.

The antioxidant properties of Antarctic Krill Oil help the body in several different ways. Together with the Omega-3, the antioxidants penetrate the fat-soluble membrane of each new cell and protect it against attacks from free radicals, which if, as we learned in Chapter 1, left alone, can deactivate the cell, damage the genetic information contained in its nucleus, damage or even destroy it. Antarctic Krill Oil protects the cellular membranes against oxidation and fortifies it so it can withstand incursions from free radicals caused by UV light, smoking, stress, the contraceptive pill and chronic diseases.

The astaxanthin contained in Antarctic Krill Oil is a particularly powerful antioxidant that acts on chronic inflammation throughout the

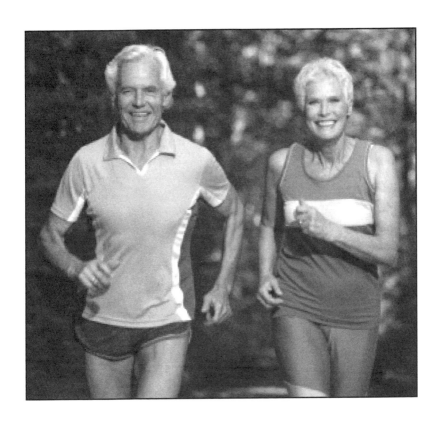

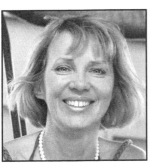

Mrs. Mary F B., 48 years old, of K. (Ref: 2495).

Premenstrual syndrome: relief from the first day

"I've suffered from premenstrual syndrome for many years. Sometimes it used to be so bad I couldn't even go about my daily business. My doctor prescribed me some medication, but it had side effects and I couldn't function normally. So, I stopped taking it. Then I decided to try Antarctic Krill Oil in the hope that it's action would be more natural. From the very first day I felt better. All my physical and emotional symptoms started to disappear. Since then, my life has changed. I wouldn't hesitate to recommend this product to any woman suffering from PMS."

body (intestines, joints, etc.). As opposed to many other antioxidants, it can also penetrate into the cells of the brain and the eye, thereby increasing its therapeutic potential. The Astaxanthin protects against the damage wrought by free radicals in the eyes (macular degeneration, cataracts), the skin cells (UV rays), the central nervous system, the blood vessels... basically every single cell in the body. It slows the aging process (we look younger) and has been proven to be effective against carpal tunnel syndrome and cardiovascular disease. Lastly, astaxanthin also protects the mucous membrane in the stomach and boosts fertility. Antarctic Krill Oil works on two fronts – anti-inflammatory and antacid – which makes it such an exceptional food supplement.

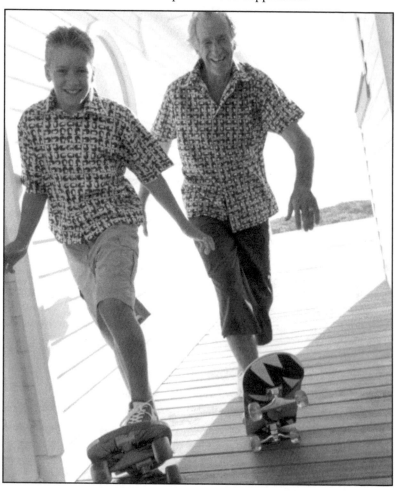

CHAPTER 3
<u>Antarctic Krill Oil as a treatment</u>

Be healthy thanks to Antarctic Krill Oil

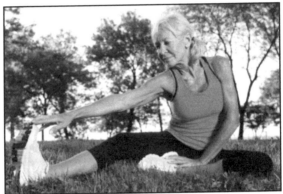

You can believe what we say, because it has now been proven in several clinical studies.

Antarctic Krill Oil boosts the healing process and can help in the following cases:

- **Premenstrual syndrome**
- **Cholesterol**
- **Arthrosis, arthritis, rheumatism and other painful joint conditions**
- **Heart attack and strokes**
- **Diabetes**

... Just to name a few (you are going to find a full list of all the other diseases in a few minutes). Antarctic Krill Oil is also excellent for your hair, your eyes, it increases your powers

The latest studies show that Antarctic Krill Oil:

Reduces Cholesterol. After just 12 weeks:
- Cholesterol reduced by 13%
- LDL reduced by 32%
- Triglycerides reduced by 11%
- Good HDL cholesterol raised by 44%

Relieves Joint Pain. After just 1 week:
- Pain reduced by 24%
- Stiffness reduced by 22%
- Flexibility increased by 16%

Prevents PMS. After just 3 months:
- Irritability reduced by 47%
- Depression reduced by 40%
- Water retention reduced by 37%
- Abdominal pain reduced by 33%

And Antarctic Krill Oil also shows great potential as a source of energy and a brain tonic and also protects the skin, fights wrinkles and more.

of concentration, combats allergies and is good for anyone who wants to increase their energy levels.

How is this possible?

What is the secret of Antarctic Krill Oil? Let's take a look at what you already know. You know that a deficiency of Omega-3 is probably your most important nutritional problem, even more so than a shortage of dietary fibre. This deficiency is one of the causes of the diseases that plague our world, touching more lives than ever. You now know that Omega-3, taken in sufficient quantity, can re-establish this balance. You also know that Omega-3 can be found in fish oil. It's not for nothing that fish oils have become the most popular and valued nutritional supplement in the world. Their preventive properties and numerous health benefits also explain why they're best sellers. Research has continued, and there's now a much better "new generation" of Omega-3, which is replacing fish oils. It's called Antarctic Krill Oil.

Antarctic Krill exceeds scientists' expectations

Antarctic Krill Oil exceeds all of scientists' expectations. Compared to fish oil supplements, it's much more effective and its potential for use in medical treatments is much greater. You now know that Antarctic Krill contains high levels of the following three high-performance nutrients:

- **Omega-3**
- **Phospholipids**
- **Powerful antioxidants**

Specialists and clinical studies have now confirmed that the synergy of these three nutrients makes Antarctic Krill Oil one of the most useful and powerful natural health products ever discovered, even for seemingly desperate health problems. Though each of these three components makes its own valuable contribution, combined together and concentrated in Antarctic Krill Oil they are even stronger!

This unique combination of ingredients in Antarctic Krill Oil contains everything we need to confront the stresses and strains so common in our modern lives.

The ingredients of Antarctic Krill

Every gram (1,000 mg) of Antarctic Krill contains approximately:

- **Phospholipid-Omega-3 complex**.................................... **400 mg**
- **Omega-3 fatty acids in total, of which:** ....**300 mg**
  EPA (eicosapentaenoic acid) **150 mg**
  and DHA (docosahexaenoic acid) **90 mg**
- **Omega-6 fatty acids, in total** ....**20 mg**
- **Omega-9 (oleic acid)** ....**70 mg**
- **Esterified astaxanthin**...**1.5 mg**
- **Vitamin A**.. **100 UI**
- **Vitamin E**.. **0.5 UI**

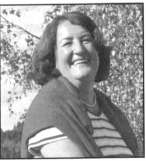

Mrs. Helen M., of F. (Ref 11034)

"My life's better now and I'm so grateful!"

"Let me just briefly say what has happened to me since I started taking Antarctic Krill Oil. During my meno-pause, I took it to allay the symptoms. It really worked well for hot flashes. But when I forgot to take it one morning, I had hot flashes the whole day. Since I've been taking Antarctic Krill Oil:

– I haven't had any more hot flashes
– I've felt much better about myself
– I have much more energy
– My skin is better and my nails are harder
– I no longer need to sleep in the afternoon – I sometimes used to have to lie down for two hours.

My life is better now, and I'm so grateful. I'm really very happy with this product."

Antarctic Krill Oil and Inflammation (CRP C-Reactive Protein)

		-40	-30	-20	-10	0	10	20	30	40
Inflammation Antarctic Krill Oil (300 mg/day)	7 days		reduced by 19.3%							
	14 days		reduced by 29.7%							
	30 days		reduced by 30.9%							
Placebo	7 days						increased by 15.7%			
	14 days						increased by 32.1%			
	30 days						increased by 25.1%			

Reduction of CRP values (inflammation values) minus 30.9% in 30 days.

Effect of Antarctic Krill Oil on Joint Pain after just 7 days:

	0	10	20	30	Reduction
Pain					Reduced by 24%
Stiffness					Reduced by 22%
Flexibility					Increased by 16%

Antarctic Krill Oil (300 mg) Relieves the Symptoms of Inflammation and Arthritis

		0	10	20	30	40
Inflammation	7 days	reduced by 19.3%				
	14 days	reduced by 29.7%				
	30 days	reduced by 30.9%				
Pain	7 days	reduced by 24.33%				
	14 days	reduced by 25.31%				
	30 days	reduced by 30.38%				
Stiffness	7 days	reduced by 21.67%				
	14 days	reduced by 28.57%				
	30 days	reduced by 26.79%				
Functional impairment	7 days	reduced by 16.02%				
	14 days	reduced by 18.21%				
	30 days	reduced by 18.13%				

Other diseases that can be effectively treated with Antarctic Krill

Premenstrual syndrome

According to specialists, between 85% and 97% of women aged under the age of 50 suffer from mild to severe pain, discomfort and mood swings every month directly caused by their menstrual cycle.

Results of Clinical Trials with Antarctic Krill Oil for Premenstrual Syndrome

Symptom		0 1 2 3 4 5 6 7	Reduction
Breast tenderness	Basic value	6.9	
	45 days	5.7	Reduced by 42%
	90 days	4.0	
Despondency	Basic value	6.7	
	45 days	5.2	Reduced by 42%
	90 days	3.9	
Stress	Basic value	7.2	
	45 days	5.7	Reduced by 38%
	90 days	4.5	
Irritability	Basic value	6.0	
	45 days	5.1	Reduced by 47%
	90 days	3.2	
Depression	Basic value	6.9	
	45 days	5.4	Reduced by 40%
	90 days	4.2	
Joint pains	Basic value	5.8	
	45 days	4.7	Reduced by 64%
	90 days	2.1	
Weight increase	Basic value	5.7	
	45 days	5.8	Reduced by 30%
	90 days	5.3	
Abdominal pain	Basic value	7.4	
	45 days	5.6	Reduced by 33%
	90 days	4.9	
Swelling	Basic value	7.6	
	45 days	5.6	Reduced by 37%
	90 days	4.8	
Flatulence	Basic value	7.6	
	45 days	6.1	Reduced by 21%
	90 days	6.0	

At least 85% of women suffer from premenstrual syndrome. It's a major cause of absence from work and relationship problems. It manifests itself in different ways in each woman and can vary from one month to the next. The symptoms are wide-ranging and unpleasant: irritability, sudden cravings (for example the desire to eat a whole box of chocolates), along with a whole range of physical symptoms: tender breasts, pain in the lower abdomen, cramps, water retention, bloating, weight gain, joint and muscular pain, tiredness and headaches.

Antarctic Krill Oil:

- Reduces abdominal pain and uterine cramps
- Reduces nausea, bloating and tiredness
- Relieves headaches, joint point and general achiness
- Lessens breast tenderness caused by premenstrual syndrome
- Combats mood swings and hunger pangs
- Helps to avoid stress, depression and tension caused by menstruation

High cholesterol

Some cholesterol reducers (such as statins) are said to be carcinogenic and can induce heart failure (because they stop the body from producing the coenzyme Q10). That's why it's important to seek out alternatives, and the Omega-3 fatty acids in Antarctic Krill Oil constitute just such a good alternative (in addition to their other benefits, mentioned at length here like, for example, reducing cholesterol and triglyceride levels). These fatty acids also provide protection against the oxidation of cholesterol and vascular deterioration. (Recommended for use with: palm oil, turmeric).

Reduction of Cholesterol: 1,000 mg Antarctic Krill Oil a Day

		0	50	100	150	200	250 Reduction
Total cholesterol	Basic value	235.83					
	90 days	204.13					reduced by 13.44%
LDL	Basic value	167.78					
	90 days	114.04					reduced by 32.03%
HDL	Basic value	57.22					
	90 days	82.35					increased by 43.92%
Triglycerides	Basic value	120.50					
	90 days	107.21					reduced by 11.03%

Maintenance dose: 500 mg Antarctic Krill Oil a Day

		0	50	100	150	200	250 Reduction
Total cholesterol	Basic value	235.83					
	180 days	192.53					reduced by 18.36%
LDL	Basic value	167.78					
	180 days	107.47					reduced by 35.94%
HDL	Basic value	57.22					
	180 days	77.71					increased by 35.81%
Triglycerides	Basic value	120.50					
	180 days	89.89					reduced by 25.40%

Vascular disease, arteriosclerosis, strokes and heart attacks

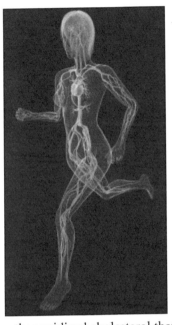

In primary and secondary prophylaxis, Antarctic Krill Oil figures among the top options for protecting the vessels and the heart. It reduces many risk factors. It slows the aggregation of thrombocytes and reduces triglyceride levels, including in menopausal women as well as lessening the risk of further narrowing of the blood vessels after a heart bypass. (Recommended for use with: palm oil capsules, grapefruit seed extract)

A sufficient intake of antioxidants is a fundamentally important factor in preventing vascular disease. They prevent the oxidation of the cholesterol, thereby attacking the root of the problem. It's not cholesterol itself, but rather oxidized cholesterol that presents a threat to the vessels.

In this regard, astaxanthin is highly effective, since it's able to

---

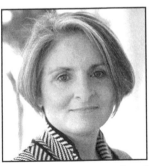

Mrs. Ruth G., of L., therapist (Ref: 14718)

"I recommend Antarctic Krill Oil with Coral Calcium..."

"I'm happy to recommend Antarctic Krill Oil with Coral Calcium, on the basis of my personal experience and that of my clients. Most of my clients who suffer from a chronic illness should take this product on a more or less long-term basis, to give it enough time to act. I particularly recommend it to people who have generalized pain to block the inflammation process. One of my patients managed to cure her tennis elbow. You should always consider every aspect of a condition. It's not enough just to treat the symptoms."

penetrate the brain. It also has an important anti-inflammatory effect. Actually, vascular diseases are basically inflammations. The anti-inflammatory action of Antarctic Krill Oil has been shown in studies on C reactive protein (an inflammation marker).

Diabetes

Thanks to its vaso-protective and anti-inflammatory properties, Antarctic Krill Oil is highly recommended in cases of diabetes, which is a condition that produces large amounts of free radicals. With Antarctic Krill Oil, there's no need to worry about developing a resistance to insulin, which would be a concern with the absorption of high doses of fish oil (3,000 mg or more).

Irregular heart beat (cardiac arrhythmia)

Antarctic Krill Oil has a beneficial effect on variations in cardiac frequency. It stabilizes the heartbeat and the neurovegetative system.

Antarctic Krill Oil looks after your heart

Another scientific study has confirmed that Antarctic Krill Oil is good for your heart. Over the course of a month, researchers followed a group of 27 patients who all suffered from hyperlipidemia (elevated levels of fat in the blood) and cardiovascular problems, giving them 1,000 mg of Antarctic Krill Oil daily, to test its effect on cholesterol and triglyceride levels.

The results of a study that we ourselves carried out showed Antarctic Krill Oil to be highly effective in the treatment of hyperlipidemia, because it causes a significant lowering of the glucose rate, total cholesterol, bad cholesterol (LDL) and triglycerides, while simultaneously increasing the good cholesterol (HDL). In this respect it's much more effective than fish oil. Taking only one 500 mg gel cap on a daily basis can maintain blood levels of glucose and lipids at a healthy level.

The results of this clinical study prove it:

After a three month period, total cholesterol was down 13%, "bad cholesterol" by 32% and triglycerides were down by 11% while "good" cholesterol had gone up 44%!

All the patients have seen an improvement in their physical functions, pain and fatigue have been reduced and they've rediscovered a much better quality of life, plus a mental, emotional and physical wellbeing.

Neurodermatitis, atopic dermatitis, (itchy, red skin)

Antarctic Krill Oil is indispensable in the treatment of these conditions, combating inflammation and supplementing treatments. (Please note that it's important to monitor intolerances carefully and get plenty of sleep; take lactobacilli (an ingredient in yogurt, cheese, chocolate and other fermented foods or as a supplement to aid intestinal function or grapefruit seed extract, for its antimycotic and antifungal properties).

Allergies

Those tested noted a reduction in seasonal allergy symptoms. This welcome secondary effect of Antarctic Krill Oil is actually because it neutralizes arachidonic acid, an allergen and inflammatory found in our food (animal fats, Omega-6). (Recommended to be taken with: MSM, Lactobacilli and/or Volcanic Minerals.)

Ulcerative colitis, Crohn's disease

The anti-inflammatory effects of Antarctic Krill Oil can be boosted by taking MSM and lactobacilli to re-establish the intestinal flora and strengthen the immune system in the case of dietary intolerance. Lactobacilli produce digestives enzymes such as proteases, lipases and lactases. Silicium has been shown to be very effective at reducing inflammation.

Migraine

Antarctic Krill Oil has been observed to reduce the frequency and intensity of migraine attacks. (Another recommendation for pressure-related cephalea: take MSM to relax the muscles. The combination of turmeric and volcanic minerals can reduce headaches associated with the liver.)

Cancer and metastasis

In the prevention of cancer, Antarctic Krill Oil reduces two risk factors: free radicals and arachidonic acid. Its powerful antioxidant capacity protects the cellular membranes against attacks from free radicals and prevents damage to the nucleus of the cell and even the formation of cancer.

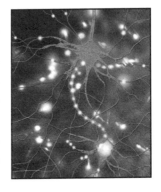

Don't forget that Antarctic Krill Oil has declared war on our diet laden in animal fats and inflammation-promoting Omega-6.

It's believed that a third of all cancers may be linked to inflammations.

People who eat a diet rich in Omega-3 are less likely to contract cancer. Experiments carried out on animals have shown it to have a retardant impact on the formation of cancers of the skin, breast, pancreas, intestine and prostate. The same effect was noted in the development of breast and intestinal cancer metastasization.

Regarding the prevention of intestinal cancer, it was noted that cellular proliferation of the mucous membrane of the intestines, which is a paraneoplastic tumour marker, responds positively. Studies with fish oil have shown that the EPA in particular slows the development of the tumours, while DHA has an anti-apoptotic action. (Recommended for use with: turmeric, silicium and/or lactobacilli.)

Psoriasis

The Inuit people, thanks to their diet rich in Omega-3 fatty acids, suffer very little psoriasis. Skin affected with psoriasis contains approximately twenty times more arachidonic acid than healthy skin. This acid triggers its well-known inflammatory reactions in the skin and joints. Fish oil can reduce the symptoms of psoriasis: the scaling, reddening or thickening of the dermis. It is also known to reduce joint pain. Studies have not yet been carried out with Antarctic Krill Oil as of yet, but it is expected to perform better than fish oil.

Multiple sclerosis

Multiple sclerosis should also be classified as an inflammatory disease. Antarctic Krill Oil can be taken in its treatment, as a supplement, to reduce inflammation.

Parkinson's disease

Parkinson's disease is primarily due to a lack of dopamine. Antarctic Krill Oil can improve dopamine levels.

Effort-induced asthma

Omega-3 fatty acids provide a beneficial treatment for this type of asthma.

Visual and cognitive faculties in babies

Pregnant women should make sure they have a sufficient intake of

Omega-3, as should breast-feeding mothers. Antarctic Krill Oil is their closest ally when it comes to boosting their baby's visual and cognitive faculties.

Macular degeneration

Macular degeneration is the result of a lack of pigments protecting the visual center. The body gets natural protection from our intake of lutein-rich green vegetables, but the problem is that we don't consume them in sufficient quantities. Astaxanthin acts in the same way as the lutein in green vegetables. We know it's present in the macula. In studies using rats, researchers at Illinois University have noted that it does indeed protect the eye. They also showed that astaxanthin, unlike zeaxanthine, doesn't form crystalline deposits in the eye. If this condition occurs, treatment with Antarctic Krill Oil may help.

Cataracts

Cataracts are caused by an agglutination of the protein fibres in the lens of the eye. This is caused by hyperglycemia (diabetes!) and free radicals. Astaxanthin, a particularly powerful antioxidant contained in Antarctic Krill Oil keeps the eyes healthy and so is a recommended treatment in the case of cataracts.

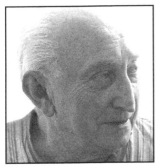

Mr. Ernest R., 82 years old of C. (Ref: 14113)

"My nerves don't bother me any more and my wife can knit again."

"My wife was born in 1933 and I was born in 1928. We discovered Antarctic Krill Oil (and Coral Calcium) about a year ago and since then we've been taking an Antarctic Krill Oil soft gel capsule and a Coral Calcium capsule every morning with breakfast. We haven't noticed any side effects. My wife, who suffered from bad arthritis in both hands and her fingers, can knit again. As for me, I had trouble with my nerves. But happily that's all in the past now. Now we can both live in happiness and harmony."

Depression and aggression

Deterioration of the cognitive functions, impulsiveness and depression are all closely linked to a low concentration of Omega-3 in the diet. Dopamine, in particular, along with serotonin (which is responsible for the subjective feeling of well-being), depends on our intake of fatty acids. Antarctic Krill Oil can prove a very effective complementary treatment.

Mobility and speech problems

Antarctic Krill Oil acts on the brain and has been proven to improve mobility and speech. Most importantly, it has even shown itself to be effective against Huntington's disease and chorea, a hereditary disease that destroys the cells of the brain and which also causes depression and aggressive states.

Childhood depression

More and more children are suffering from depression. A scientific study was carried out on twenty depressed children, in which ten children were given an Omega-3 supplement while others received a placebo.

After a few weeks, the children who had been given the Omega-3 were clearly feeling much better, while the other group were not. Antarctic Krill Oil contains valuable Omega-3 and is ideal as a supplement to a medical course of treatment.

Did you know?

FACT#1: 11,737 scientific research reports at the U.S. National Library all have one thing in common: Omega-3 and its effects on your health!

FACT#2: Three large controlled studies of 32,000 participants prove that Omega-3 supplements reduce cardiovascular events by 19% to 45%!

This is unquestionable evidence.

CHAPTER 4
<u>Could Antarctic Krill Oil even be used to treat cancer?</u>

The importance of Omega-3 in the treatment of cancer and other serious diseases

You know now that Omega-3 fatty acids have a considerable prophylactic effect. This is particularly true for cardiovascular conditions and chronic degenerative diseases (joint deterioration). A connection has even been found between a deficiency of Omega-3 in the tissue and an increase in neurodegenerative disease and mental illness.

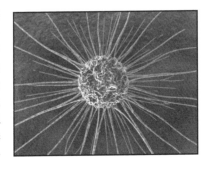

A study carried out at Pittsburgh University (USA), showed that two types of Omega-3 fatty acids are effective in the prevention and treatment of cancer: EPA (eicosapentaenoic acid) and DHA (docosahexaenoic acid).

These Omega-3 fatty acids not only prevent the proliferation of cancer cells, they also cause them to die (apoptosis). Regular absorption of these two active ingredients inhibits beta-catenin, a protein active in the development of various tumours.

The research team at the British Paterson Institute for Cancer Research, at Manchester University in England, published an article in the British Journal of Cancer that DHA and EPA were also effective in the treatment of pancreatic cancer.

The scientists Bergstrom, Samuelsson and Vane received a Nobel Prize several years ago, for showing that Omega-3 deficiency can trigger the onset of various diseases. Since then, we've discovered that two groups of elcosanoids, play an essential role in regulating blood pressure, kidney function, the immune system, cell division and combating pain. Other elcosanoids activate the aggregation of blood platelets and help blood coagulation.

Antarctic Krill Oil contains Omega-3

An article which appeared in the journal Nutrition and Cancer describes the treatment of a lung cancer in its initial stages through the absorption, over a three-year period, of a daily dosage of 15 grams of Omega-3 fatty acids together with various other nutritional supplements (while at the same time avoiding any foods rich in Omega-6). The treatment was recommended by a professor in biochemistry, Ron Pardini, of Reno University (Nevada, USA). He specializes in the study of Omega-3 and has proven that, in rats at least, Omega-3 fatty acids significantly inhibit the growth of cancer cells in the breasts, ovaries, colon, prostate and pancreas.

So we can see that Omega-3 fatty acids are useful in the prevention and treatment of many diseases (although of course you need to maintain the balance between Omega-3 and Omega-6).

But how did we arrive at the conclusion of a possible link between Omega-6 and cancer?

A brief look back

In 1923, American scientists Burr and Evans discovered that rats that didn't eat any foods with unsaturated fatty acids got ill. They concluded that essential fatty acids were fundamentally important for good health. Evans gave a name to these polyunsaturated fatty acids: vitamin F. Later, Burr showed there were two fatty acids: Omega-3 (alpha-linoleic acid) and Omega-6 (linoleic acid).

It wasn't until the 1970's that the link between Omega-3 and cardiovascular disease was finally established: A Danish epidemiologist noted that it was because of the Omega-3 in fish that the Inuit didn't suffer from cardiovascular problems.

He reached this conclusion by observing how the Inuit people only suffered heart attacks if they left their country and changed their traditional eating habits.

When you consider that the Inuit people are big consumers of Omega-3, which they get from fish, seals and whales, this is a logical enough conclusion.

Further studies have confirmed this. Inhabitants of Crete have a diet extremely rich in Omega-3, which is said to be the reason for their very long life expectancy. The longevity of the Japanese is also attributed to their high consumption of Omega-3 (as you saw on the graph on page 29).

Over the course of years, the hypothesis of the benefits of Omega-3 continued to expand, not only with regards to cardiovascular disease, but also chronic joint conditions and cancer. We now know that a minimal deficiency of Omega-3 in the tissue can trigger the onset of neurodegenerative disease and mental illness.

It's incontestable that cancer is less common among people who consume high proportions of seafood. This is logical, since seafood contains long-chain Omega-3 polyunsaturates.

The Japanese eat a lot of fish and have a very low incidence of cancer. Men who eat a fish-rich diet have a lower risk of contracting prostate cancer. The same is true of cancers of the stomach and intestines. When the majority of your food intake is fish, these diseases appear less frequently. Eating a diet rich in Omega-3 helps to reduce certain hormones that appear in high levels in patients with cancer. Even chemotherapy is more effective on patients whose diet includes a significant amount of Omega-3. The properties of Omega-3 can be proven in medical tests. And that's just the beginning…

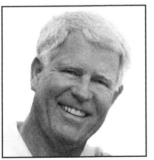

Mr. Rodolph L., 68 years old of S. (Ref: 10758)

"In better shape intellectually and more flexible and with greater stamina!"

"I'd particularly like to talk about Antarctic Krill Oil. After just a short time, my mind and body were in better form, I felt more supple and had more stamina. I never get colds anymore. I'm 68 years old and still play sports. As a writer, I'm particularly grateful for the improvement it made to my brainpower. I'm grateful to nature for giving us this powerful fountain of youth in the form of Antarctic Krill Oil."

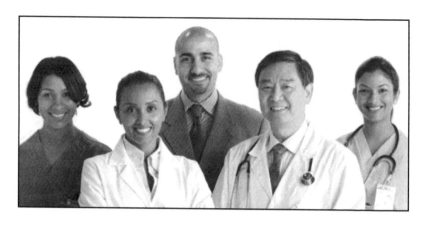

Liver Cancer

At a conference of the American Association for Cancer Research, in Washington, representatives from Pittsburgh University presented a study that showed that Omega-3 DHA and EPA could provide an effective treatment not only for preventing, but also for treating liver cancer.

On the same subject, Doctor Tong Wu, of the Transplant Pathology Department at Pittsburgh University Medical School, wrote: *"We have known for some time that Omega-3 could inhibit certain cancer cells. That's why we want to know if these substances are also capable of inhibiting cancer cells in the liver and, if so, how do they do it."*

Researchers started by observing the effect of Omega-3 and Omega-6 polyunsaturates on hepatocellular carcinoma, which are responsible for between 80 and 90 percent of liver cancer types and usually cause death within three to six months of diagnosis. They treated the cancer cells for 12 to 48 hours with EPA and DHA of the Omega-3 series, plus arachidonic acid of the Omega-6 series.

They soon saw that both DHA and EPA (Omega-3) halted the growth of the cancer-producing cells, depending on the dose, while arachidonic acid (Omega-6) did not give any significant results.

In addition, treatment with DHA and EPA reduced levels of a protein known as beta-catenin, which plays a major role in the growth of various tumours.

Doctor Wu explained it as follows: *"Beta-catenin promotes cell growth and also plays a part in the proliferation of cancer cells. With our discovery, that Omega-3 can reduce beta-catenin levels, we have clearly proven that these composites have the capacity to interfere, in many different circumstances, in the progression of the tumour."*

Researchers treated a cholangiocarcinoma (a particularly aggressive liver tumor) for 12 to 48 hours with Omega-3 or with Omega-6 (this type of cancer is very rare and is usually fatal).

Treatment with DHA and EPA fatty acids inhibited the growth of the cancer cells, while treatment with arachidonic acid, of the Omega-6 series showed no effect. In this case too, treatment with DHA triggered a sort of division of the PARP in the cells of the cholangiocarcinoma. And treatment with the DHA and EPA significantly reduced beta-catenin levels.

In conclusion, Omega-3 may be considered an effective treatment for liver cancer. They can also protect against non-alcoholic steatohepatitis, a disease caused by high levels of fat in the liver that can, in the worst case, lead to cirrhosis or liver cancer. Antarctic Krill Oil may be an ideal cure in such cases.

Prostate Cancer

A British team of researchers from the famous Paterson Institute for Cancer Research, at Manchester University, published a study in the British Journal of Cancer, that concluded that a diet rich in Omega-3 could prevent benign prostate cancer developing into an aggressive cancer.

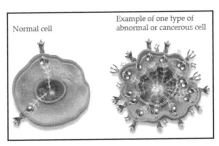

Normal cell   Example of one type of abnormal or cancerous cell

The researchers based their conclusion on the fact that prostate cancer really becomes dangerous when the cancer cells infiltrate other tissues, located outside the prostate, for example the bone marrow. Omega-3 can prevent this from happening.

Scientists have studied the action of Omega-3 and Omega-6 on prostate cancer cells and reached the conclusion that Omega-6 promoted the formation of cancer cells in the bone marrow, while Omega-3 prevented it.

In summary:

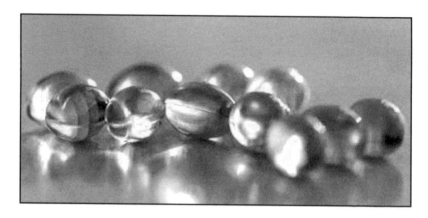

Omega-3 fatty acids can be useful in the prophylaxis and treatment of cancer, particularly cancer of the liver, pancreas, lungs and prostate.

Omega-3 fatty acids thin the blood, while Omega-6 fatty acids promote the formation of clots. This is important to know if you have heart or circulation problems. It's important to make sure you take in the right quantities of these two fatty acids.

The problem is that we currently eat too much Omega-6. To re-establish the balance, you should increase your Omega-3 intake.

Omega-3 fatty acids play a fundamental role in the process of inflammation, the regulation of blood flow, the control of ionic transport and the modulation of synaptic transmission. They are cancer inhibitors.

Omega-3 fatty acids are useful in the prevention and treatment of cancer of the liver and pancreas.

So, here is our conclusion:

Supplementing your diet with Omega-3 may have a positive impact on the diseases we've mentioned and their prevention.

Omega-3 fatty acids are fundamental components of Antarctic Krill Oil. The absorption of Antarctic Krill Oil has many long-term health benefits and could ultimately provide amazing results in the treatment of cancers.

Antarctic Krill Oil benefits:

Antarctic Krill Oil can maintain long-term health and support the treatment and healing process of the following diseases:

- **Arthrosis, arthritis, rheumatism and other joint diseases**
- **High cholesterol, hyperlipoproteinemia**
- **Vascular disease, arteriosclerosis, strokes (aneurysm) and heart attack**
- **Diabetes**
- **Heart arrhythmia**
- **Psoriasis, neurodermatitis, atopic dermatitis and other skin disorders**

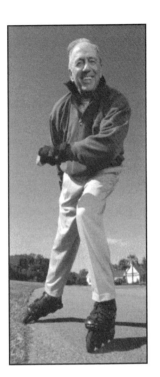

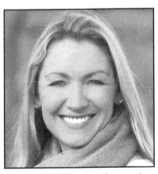

Mrs. Yvonne S., 31 years old of Z. (Ref: 19560)

Bunions, knee problems, painful periods... Antarctic Krill helps!

"My father-in-law, who's 63, introduced me to this product. He had a large bunion that disappeared thanks to Antarctic Krill Oil and Coral Calcium. He told me he also got new found energy. My mother, who's 62, had had a large growth on her foot for years which finally went away and the rheumatism she suffered in her knee had faded to almost nothing. I myself am 31 with two children and I also take Antarctic Krill Oil and Coral Calcium. Since I started taking it, I no longer get painful periods. This product helps, that's clear."

- Allergies and asthma
- Ulcerous colitis and Crohn's disease
- Migraines
- Premenstrual syndrome and menstrual pain
- Colon, liver, prostate, breast cancer and other types of cancers and metastasis
- Multiple sclerosis
- Parkinson's disease
- Alzheimer's disease
- Visual and cognitive problems in babies
- Macular degeneration
- Cataracts
- Depression and aggressivity
- ADHD (attention deficit and hyperactvity disorder)
- Bipolar disorder and schizophrenia
- Mobility and speech problems
- Childhood depression

Supplementing your diet with Omega-3 fatty acids may have a positive impact on these diseases and their prevention.

Omega-3 fatty acids are fundamental components of Antarctic Krill Oil.

The absorption of Antarctic Krill Oil can have long-lasting health benefits and could ultimately give incredible results in the treatment of cancers.

Various clinical studies have proven that Antarctic Krill Oil...

- Is a powerful anti-inflammatory
- Has an antioxidant capacity 300 times higher than vitamins A and E and 48 times higher than the Omega-3 in fish oils,

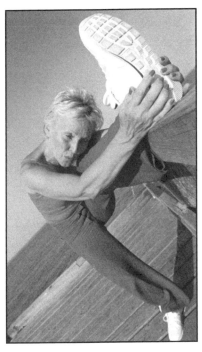

which are already powerful antioxidants!

– Reduces inflammation, pain and joint discomfort in cases of arthritis, osteoarthritis and other joint conditions.

– Helps prevent and treat cardio-vascular disease by reducing inflammation and keeping lipid levels in the bloodstream within a healthy range.

– Reduces levels of glucose, "bad" cholesterol and tri-glycerides while at the same time increasing levels of "good" cholesterol

– Relieves physical and emo-tional premenstrual symptoms

– Contributes to the proper functioning of the organs and tissue

– Prevents the damage caused by free radicals

– Improves general health, vitality and overall wellbeing

One gram (1,000 mg) of Antarctic Krill contains 300 mg of Omega-3 fatty acids, of which 150 mg is EPA (very important for the proper functioning of the immune system) and 90 mg of DHA (vital for good brain function). Antarctic Krill also contains omega fatty acid types 6 and 9.

Antarctic Krill regulates and improves cardiovascular fun-ction, blood glucose levels, energy production, liver function and physical performance. It relieves the symptoms of PMS and reduces joint aches and pains.

Antarctic Krill Oil is 100% pure nature

Antarctic Krill Oil is a natural extract. So what we are offering here is a 100% natural product that is both outstandingly effective

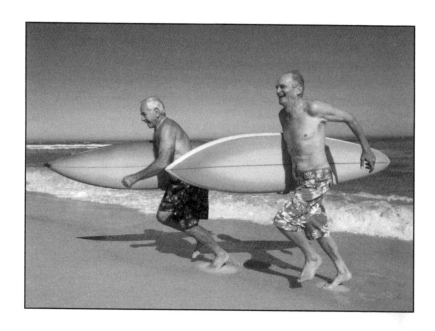

and capable of providing us with everything we need to deal with the stresses and strains of modern life. Your brain needs specific substances (different types of phospholipids) to manage or reduce stress. Antarctic Krill Oil contains these substances.

Thanks to its high Omega-3 content, Antarctic Krill Oil has a dual preventive and curative effect.

The antioxidants contained in Antarctic Krill Oil slow the aging process. You stay young and dynamic for longer.

The anti-inflammatory action of Antarctic Krill Oil can also, for example, prevent heart attacks. Penguins and the majority of the Inuit people don't get heart attacks specifically because of the large quantities of Omega-3 they eat daily, the vital elements of which are also contained in Antarctic Krill Oil soft gel capsules.

Even women who suffer from pre-menstrual syndrome find Antarctic Krill Oil a precious ally in the natural regulation of the hormonal system.

Antarctic Krill also gives protection against UV rays, thereby preventing malignant melanoma (skin cancer).

Antarctic Krill Oil can be used in many different treatments as well as prevention, for: arthrosis, arthritis, rheumatism, high cholesterol, basically all inflammatory diseases and painful joint conditions, etc... And it's also been proven to be effective in many types of cancers.

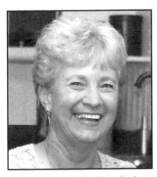

Mrs. Amalia S, of G.
(Ref: 14874)

Chronic polyarthritis

"I've suffered from polyarthritis for thirty-eight years. I get it in my hands, which are now quite deformed. Recently, I came across a leaflet about Antarctic Krill Oil with Coral Calcium. It said this product could also help reduce excess acidity. I'd always known my condition was linked to my diet, so I ordered a treatment of Antarctic Krill Oil soft gel capsules and Coral Calcium capsules. After just five days, I could feel the first benefits. Since discovering it, I've taken Antarctic Krill Oil and Coral Calcium regularly. I don't even try to understand why it works so well, all I know is that it really works on inflammation and excess acidity.

I had been taking cortisone tablets for twenty years, to the point where I was taking 1 mg doses. I haven't taken it since last year, because the attacks have been getting less and less frequent since I've been taking Antarctic Krill Oil and Coral Calcium. And, for a few months now, I haven't suffered from polyarthritis at all.

I'm aware that I'm 78 years old so, when I do the gardening or the housework, I know my hands aren't as strong as they used to be. But I can't really say I have any pain. Basically, I'm happy. I go for walks in the forest, usually in the mornings. In the afternoons, I do some work in the garden. I'm grateful I can still do my own housework."

Conclusion

To conclude, we can now affirm that Antarctic Krill Oil combined with Coral Calcium are Mother Nature's ultimate remedies of the 21st Century to prevent and cure many of the most common diseases, to feel younger, more energetic and dynamic – Mother Nature's latest secrets for a longer and much healthier life.

> **Antarctic Krill Oil and Coral Calcium are two products that come to us directly from Mother Nature.**
>
> **Antarctic Krill Oil soft gel capsules and Okinawa Coral Calcium capsules: a perfect balance of carefully chosen ingredients bring a natural wonder within your reach.**
>
> **What more could you ask for?**

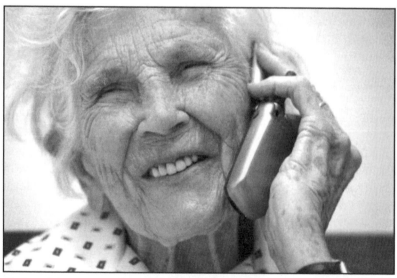

Today, it's proven that a small daily supply of Antarctic Krill Oil combined with Coral Calcium can protect you against the most common diseases and really improve your health to help you stay healthy and active until a very advanced age.